It's Okay to Be Me

A Journey to God's Heart by Way of Cancer

Veronica Arnold

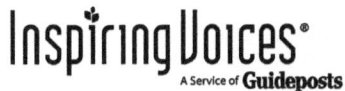

Inspiring Voices®

A Service of **Guideposts**

Inspiring Voices books may be ordered through booksellers or by contacting:

Inspiring Voices
1663 Liberty Drive
Bloomington, IN 47403
www.inspiringvoices.com
1-(866) 697-5313

Because of the dynamic nature of the Internet, any web addresses or links contained in this book may have changed since publication and may no longer be valid. The views expressed in this work are solely those of the author and do not necessarily reflect the views of the publisher, and the publisher hereby disclaims any responsibility for them.

Any people depicted in stock imagery provided by Thinkstock are models, and such images are being used for illustrative purposes only.

Certain stock imagery © Thinkstock.

ISBN: 978-1-4624-0408-7 (sc)
ISBN: 978-1-4624-0407-0 (e)

Library of Congress Control Number: 2012920813

Printed in the United States of America

Inspiring Voices rev. date: 11/5/2012

"An amazing, inspirational and life-changing account of a personal journey. Veronica's words are so vivid I can picture her telling me her story as if in conversation with each other over coffee. Veronica has given a gift to others by sharing her story."

—Ashley Hood, medical/oncology social worker

To three great ladies who have profoundly influenced my life:

My mother, Mary Schneider, who built into me a solid foundation of absolute trust in the truth of God's Word (now deceased);

My stepmother, Evelyn Porter, who demonstrated to me the inestimable value of a calm, practical approach to life (now deceased); and

My mother-in-law, Earline Zook, who modeled for me a beautiful way to grow old. Her good humor, zest for life, unwavering faith in God, and acceptance of the realities of aging have created a path for me to follow as I approach the later years of my life.

And to my husband, Jerry Arnold, whom God has used as an anchor for my soul on the stormy sea of life.

Psalm 28:7
The Lord is my strength and my shield;
my heart trusts in him, and I am helped.
My heart leaps for joy
and I will give thanks to him in song.

Nahum 1:7
The Lord is good,
a refuge in times of trouble.
He cares for those who trust in him.

Contents

Preface

In 2007, I took a two-year biblical counseling course from Re-Connect Ministries in Greeley, Colorado, that rocked my world. I had been a Christian and involved in good churches for fifty-five years, but I learned things in that course that I had never heard in church. The sovereignty of God, for example, was explored in great depth. My mouth hung open for several months. I kept thinking, *This can't be right*, but it was what Scripture said, so it had to be right. Rather than me being in control of my life, as I had previously thought, I learned that God has absolute rule over all creation. He has the right and power to do anything He wants in my life to accomplish His purpose, which is to see Jesus more perfectly formed in my life.

When I was finally able to accept that God knows what He is doing, He has a plan, and He is working His plan, I felt an immense comfort. I had been like a cork bouncing along on the ocean, feeling at the top of a wave when I succeeded at something but at the bottom of the trough when I failed. Now I knew that, regardless of my circumstances, I was right on track. I was precisely where God wanted me to be in order to learn the lessons He had for me. While He certainly makes me responsible for my choices, I am not powerful enough to screw up His plan for me. All I have to do is trust Him. While I had always trusted as much as I knew of Him, this understanding gave me a new sense of stability. The old hymn was right. All I had to do was "Trust and Obey."

Equally important was an emerging understanding of my own identity. I began to realize that people's identities—who they believe they are—are absolutely critical to solving most of the issues that trouble them. If I believe I am a screw-up, then I will screw up most things I attempt. If I believe I am a child of the King, I will walk out the truth of who He created me to be. I learned that God created me from the beginning as a precious and perfect jewel. It is true that I have been dipped in the mud of sin, but His blood has wiped me clean so I can shine again, reflecting His light. To the extent that I believe this, I will live a purposeful, fulfilled life.

My belief that God loved me made changes in my spirit from the moment I asked Jesus into my heart at age six, but my emotions didn't seem to be affected so much. Although I knew deep in my born-again spirit that I was infinitely valuable to God, I felt rejected by people, and I shut down my emotions. As I studied the material for the biblical counseling course much later, and in the years since that time, God revealed to me lies I had believed and replaced them with His truth. This book is the story of the way my cancer journey was the crowning jewel on top of a lifetime of God calling me to Him that helped me see it really is okay to be me.

You don't have to be from a horribly dysfunctional family in order to grow up believing lies that keep you from receiving the unbounded love of God. People from the most stable home environments do. The Bible tells us that at the moment of conversion, we die and God recreates us to look just like Jesus. That new, born-again spirit wants only to please God. But indwelling sin is still present in our bodies—a force separate from us whose intense mission, 24/7, is to do everything it can to make us feel separate from God and all the joy He has for us. When we learn that the enemy is *not* us, we can begin to fight a winning battle. We can begin to reckon ourselves dead to sin's lies and be alive only to God.[1]

Being alive only to God equals being alive only to love, because God is love. Any message that is opposed to "I am loved" can be traced to indwelling sin and its lies. As you read this book, I hope you will see a picture of what that battle can look like and how it can be won.

---

1   See Romans 6:11.

Acknowledgements

I owe an enormous debt of gratitude to a few friends who have helped me craft this book. In 2012 I took a Creative Nonfiction Writing class at Front Range Community College. My teacher, Kerri Mitchell, and my classmates gave me honest critiques and great ideas for improvement. My friends Sally Graham and Harry Black also helped with valuable feedback about technical issues. My sincere thanks to all of you.

Chapter 1

I Placed My Hand in His

"It's cancer," my doctor told me over the phone, choking up, devastated. It was July 22, 2011. Earlier, he had diagnosed the little lump in my breast as only a cyst, nothing to be concerned about, but now …

I was not devastated. Rather, I felt like a warrior emerging from months-long training to engage in battle. When I told my sister the news, she seemed confused. "I hear the words you are saying," she said, "but the tone of your voice doesn't match. Are you *happy* about this?" She didn't understand my "warrior" voice.

The previous three months had been boot-camp training for this daunting challenge, though I had not known it at the time. In April, our pastor told his leadership team to begin studying what the Bible said about spiritual warfare. I put the two passages[2] he mentioned on my list of verses to memorize, and I repeated them aloud five times a day. My attention was drawn to Ephesians 6:13 (New International Version): "Therefore put on the full armor of God, so that when the day of evil comes, you may be able to stand your ground, and after you have done everything, to stand." One word flashed like a neon light as I meditated on this verse. *When* the day of evil comes. Not *if* but *when*. The day of evil would come. I could count on that. The only question was this: would I stand firm, fully protected by God's armor?

---

2   2 Corinthians 10:3–6 and Ephesians 6:10–18.

This thought, that the day of evil would certainly come, did not engender fear in me. I simply mulled it over, letting it become a fact of my worldview. It changed the level of my expectations. If I expected life to be without a fight, then I would indeed be devastated by something like a cancer diagnosis. It's not that my outlook became grim, expecting any moment to receive bad news. Rather, I realized that standing in the fire with God[3] is a much safer place to be than abandoning His presence in an attempt to avoid the flames. The temptation is always to try to hide from the truth that He insists upon making clear to me. I am wrongly inclined to believe that worrying about my situation will be much more effective than running to Him for protection and provision.

Thirty-two years earlier, my husband, Jerry, and I had become involved with what is known as "the faith message"—a teaching in the Christian church that if you truly love God, you will be able to stay free of all sickness and disease by simply rebuking it in the name of Jesus and commanding it to be gone. In the last six years, I had learned about and surrendered to God's sovereignty—His right and power to do anything He wants in my life in order to mold me more surely into the image of Jesus. I still believed in God's power and desire to heal our bodies, but now my focus was on letting Jesus live His life in me.

My Western civilization class at Front Range Community College had ended May 5, about two months before my cancer diagnosis. I don't normally do well without structure, so the long summer break between classes always challenged me.

This summer wasn't as bad as previous summers, however. My husband, Jerry, had finally decided that his left knee hurt badly enough to have knee-replacement surgery on May 23. After his surgery, I had

---

3   A reference to the story in Daniel 3:13–27 of the three Israelite captives who were thrown into the fiery furnace for worshipping God rather than King Nebuchadnezzar's image. When the king looked into the furnace, he saw four men there, and one of them was the Son of God. When they brought the three Israelites out of the furnace, they were not burned and didn't even smell like smoke.

six weeks of full-time work helping him numerous times a day with various exercises. This added a welcome focus to my daily routine. I had started a diet and was losing weight. I had taken my trusty bike down from the garage wall and was cycling a few times a week and loving it. I felt great!

On Wednesday, July 13, I went to my doctor for my annual physical exam. As usual, he pronounced me healthy as a horse. He did find one small lump near the nipple of my left breast, but he was sure it was only a cyst and nothing to worry about. Nevertheless, just to be sure, he sent me to the Breast Diagnostic Center for a mammogram and an ultrasound the following Monday. I felt the beginnings of a premonition that everything might not be right.

On the way home from that physical exam, I noticed the signboard of a church near our house. The message for the week was, "I will fear no evil, for God is with me." I remembered the entire verse from Psalm 23 (NIV), "Even though I walk through the valley of the shadow of death, I will fear no evil for you are with me; your rod and your staff, they comfort me." The valley of the shadow[4] of death suddenly became a distinct possibility for me, but at the same time, God's presence became even more real. *Because* He is with me, I will fear no evil while I walk through that valley. I noticed that it doesn't say "I *need* fear no evil" but "I *will* fear no evil." This absence of fear was a certainty as long as I kept my attention focused on God's presence with me.

Although there would be challenges ahead, I had sunk my roots deep into the soil of God's promises and His presence in my life. I was not afraid. In fact, I was pumped. Here was a chance for God to roll up His sleeves and show Himself strong on my behalf. *Bring it on!* I thought.

The ultrasound revealed two masses in my left breast. The doctor who explained the significance of the ultrasound told me, "There are masses like that which are benign." I thought at the time that he was

---

4   Not the valley of *death* but the valley of the *shadow* of death. *Shadow*, I believe in this
     context, is tantamount to fear. As Christians, whether or not death is imminent, we
     need not fear it.

3

trying to tell me as gently as possible that they were quite possibly *not* benign. I was amazed and thankful for his considerate way of pointing me in the direction of that possibility.

On Wednesday, I went in for a biopsy on both of those masses. Medical professionals put in two tiny titanium chips at the site of the biopsies so the masses could be easily found in the future. "Aha!" I later gloated to my husband, Mr. Titanium Knee. "You're not the only one with bionics!"

On Friday, Jerry and I drove to Red Feather Lakes, a small mountain town about fifty miles west of us, to pick up my brother-in-law, Rodney, who had been attending a weeklong retreat. My sister, Bethany, had been at our house all that time participating in a national Frisbee competition.

When we got back into cell phone range late in the morning, there was a message on my phone from my doctor, asking me to call him. I knew that was not good news. Doctors don't personally call you with *good* news. Of course, I had to leave a message for him to call me and then wait several hours for him to do so. During that time, I was tempted to begin thinking of all the cancer words—*mastectomy, chemo, radiation,* and so on. But I knew where that path would lead, and I was not willing to go there. I would have to consider those options soon enough, but for the moment I asked the Lord for something else to think about. Soon I was humming a song and praising Him for the beautiful day.

Later that afternoon the doctor called back. "It's cancer," he said, choking up. "I'm so sorry."

Giving him a chance to collect himself, I asked, "What is the next step?"

"I'll book an appointment for you with the surgeon, and you can talk to him. There are several options for the surgery itself, and he will explain all that to you. Are you ok?"

"I'm fine," I said. "God is with me. I have nothing to fear."

My pastor's sermon on the following Sunday was tailor-made for my situation. The title was "There's a Hole in the Bucket." Pastor Rick's point was that if we have faith in God only when we feel on top of our game, then that's a leaky bucket. Our faith has to be in God the promise-giver and His promises in every situation, good or bad— never in our own strength or faith. This was good news for me. In the bewildering maze of my journey, I would not have to stay on top of my game. Regardless of my feelings, I could trust that God's promises were true and that He would be utterly faithful to see me through. I didn't have to fight cancer or bury my head under my pillow to escape the process. I just needed to turn to God.

I placed my hand in His, took a deep breath, and stepped into His provision with an exhilarating sense of anticipation. I knew Jesus lived in me, and I asked Him to express His life in my thoughts, my emotions, my words, and my actions.

Chapter 2

The Lie: I Am Not Lovable

I had not always been so confident in God's promises. Although I had believed the Bible's truth from the time I was a small child, for many years there had been a disconnect between what I believed in my mind and the way I felt in my heart. When my mother's divorce and remarriage brought feelings of abandonment and rejection, I built a wall to keep people at arm's length. My mother's leniency in my formative years only added to my sense of inadequacy. Polar differences in the way my husband and I viewed life reinforced my feelings of rejection. It was only when God began to teach me how to dismantle my wall and connect with people that I began to experience a gut-level trust in His work in my life that created a joyful acceptance of my own value.

My mom and dad divorced when I was too young to remember them being together. Mom remarried when I was four, convincing herself she loved Albert long enough to marry him and become pregnant with their daughter, my sister, Gail. By that time, my mother realized she didn't love him after all. She was not willing to hurt him the way she had hurt my father by leaving him, so she stayed with Albert until he died some forty years later.

When she explained all this to me in my early teenage years, I understood why my mother had left my father, even though she loved him (she didn't know how to handle his violent temper), and why she married Albert and stayed with him (he had a house and a steady job and she had two children she couldn't support on her own). But that understanding couldn't change the pattern of rejection that had already been set in motion.

My best friend in my preschool years lived in the house across the street from ours. Besides playing together, we sometimes spent the night at each other's houses. When I stayed at her home, the interaction between her parents fascinated me. They kissed each other good-bye. *Hmm*, I thought. *I wonder why my parents don't kiss good-bye.*

One morning I carefully watched as Albert was leaving to go to work. Just as I had suspected, he didn't kiss Mom good-bye. Before Albert closed the door behind him, I boldly spoke up. "Mom, why don't you kiss Daddy good-bye like Darlene's mom kisses her daddy?" Mom and Albert looked at each other and with a great deal of discomfort gave each other a perfunctory peck before he escaped.

This didn't really satisfy me, but unwilling to reproduce that kind of discomfort, I let it slide and didn't mention it again. It was obvious that my mom and Albert didn't enjoy the kind of love that was supposed to live in a marriage. Although they never displayed overt affection for each other, they never seemed to fight and they presented a united front regarding the everyday issues of life. Each performed the necessary functions of running a household and raising kids, but there was never any hugging or kissing or enjoying each other.

This absence of love between them made it hard for me to feel in my heart the love I knew my mom felt for me. She stayed home and took good care of my older brother Don (four years my senior) and me, and later our little sister Gail (seven years my junior), and the house. She was a good person, although she harbored a certain cynicism when it came to men. Her first marriage to the love of her life hadn't worked because of his temper; and she was not happy with Albert. I soaked up that cynicism well, and its accompanying sarcasm colored my life for many years to come.

When I was five, some friends came to our house and explained

God's plan of salvation to Mom and Albert, who received God's gift of eternal life. We began attending a church in La Porte, a big city about ten miles from our tiny hometown of Union Mills, Indiana. During the days, Mom listened to a Christian radio station that featured devotional messages and Christian music. When she wasn't listening to the radio, she was humming. Although her marriage was less than what she'd always hoped for, she found an inner spring of joy in her walk with God. She taught Sunday school, memorized Scripture, and taught us to memorize Scripture. She made sure our family gathered every night to read a chapter from the Bible and kneel by our chairs to pray.

Albert was also a good person. His mother had emigrated from Germany and spoke with such a thick accent that I could hardly understand her when we went to visit her farm about half an hour away. Albert was a hard worker. He had built our house himself; he maintained a huge garden and raised chickens, rabbits, and ducks; and for his entire career, he was the janitor at our school. This involved going to work at 3 a.m. in order to stoke the coal furnace that heated the building, coming home for breakfast, and then going back to work until sometime in the afternoon. When I went to school, it was actually a point of pride for me that my dad was the janitor. Don, Gail, and I were the only students in the whole entire school who were allowed in the furnace room—sometimes we had to fetch Dad from there if he was needed for an emergency cleanup.

In later years, when I was thirteen, we began attending the tiny Baptist church in our town. Albert donated two-thirds of his huge garden plot so the church could have its own building and parsonage rather than renting rooms downtown. In addition to his job and taking care of the rest of the garden, he also spent every afternoon and evening working on the church property next door. He spent his downtime at home reading the newspaper or his Bible or watching TV. The man never took a nap that I knew of. Although he liked to be busy with something, he was not driven to make a name for himself. He was kind to the neighbors and enjoyed shooting the breeze with friends.

Albert was a tolerable father for my older brother Don and me, but he was not affectionate, and I desperately needed affection from him. When I was a very small child, for example, I tried to sit on his lap. That lasted for only a few minutes before he said, "I can't have you on my lap. My leg was hurt in the war, and it hurts to have you sit on it."

I understood that and decided to be content just snuggling up next to him. "I can't really do that either," he said. Even at that age, I could tell a brush-off when I saw it, and my learned cynicism kicked in. I felt rejected and in turn built a wall against him. I looked for things to detest about him in order to prove my wall was necessary.

For example, Albert had an annoying habit of sniffing. About the time I got home from school and began to practice piano, he also got home from work and sat in his chair in the same room to read his paper. He would rattle the paper and sniff, especially if I hit a wrong note. I never said anything about the way that annoyed me, but I seethed inside. Maybe that's one reason I was not eager to practice and didn't take lessons for very long.

My real father was absent most of the time simply because he and my mother were divorced. This absence felt like abandonment to me, and because children think they are the center of the universe, I subconsciously believed it was because I was somehow flawed. I spent most of my life crying out, "What is wrong with me? Somebody tell me, so I can fix it!" But nobody ever did. At the same time, even though I felt flawed, I knew I was worth loving because I knew in my spirit that God loved me. This understanding had begun when I received God's gift of eternal life at the age of six.

I don't ever remember not going to church regularly. Sunday morning, Sunday night, and Wednesday night services were the minimum services we attended weekly. We were there every time the doors opened. Each service required a ten-mile drive from our small town to La Porte and back. I did not imagine that life should be any other way.

The summer after my sixth birthday, a gospel magician came to the Baptist church in Union Mills, where we would later become members, for a series of services. He used his magic tricks to illustrate that there were two places people could go after they died: heaven or hell. Heaven was the good, desirable place, and hell was the bad place—you definitely wanted to avoid that. There was only one way to get to heaven, and that was to ask Jesus to live in your heart.

One night the gospel magician spent the night at our house. After supper, I tugged on Mom's arm when she came into my room. "Mom," I whispered, "I want to ask Jesus into my heart."

"That's great, honey," she said. "I'll tell the magician and he can help you."

She conferred with the magician and then gathered Albert and my brother, Don, in the living room. That room was actually two rooms with an arch across the ceiling between them. On that evening, the couch was in the middle of the two rooms, facing the front of the house. Behind the couch were a dining room table pushed up against a wall and an upright piano against the wall that divided the living room from the kitchen. The TV faced the couch, and there were two chairs and lamps in that section of the room.

The magician took charge of the situation. "Your mom tells me you want to ask Jesus into your heart. Is that right?" he asked.

I nodded. "You said I had to do that if I wanted to go to heaven, didn't you?"

"That's right," he agreed.

"Well, I do."

"I'm glad to hear that," he said. "Let's all kneel here by the couch and chairs, and I will lead you in a prayer. Would that be okay?"

"Yes," I said.

After we were all settled in our kneeling positions, the magician said a prayer, one phrase at a time, giving me time to repeat the phrases after him. Then he welcomed me into the family of God.

There were no fireworks at that conversion, and nothing felt

11

different. But I believed God's promises were true, and I knew I was now His child forever.

Seven years later, by the age of thirteen, I had become miserable. Our church emphasized all the sinful things you must not do, such as wear makeup, dance, or go to the movies. I didn't have a problem with all that; I believed those things were sinful and I wanted nothing to do with them. However, that austere lifestyle made it extremely difficult for a person my age to have friends. I was the only one in my school who lived that way. There was very little in my life that attracted friendships. Therefore, I was lonely. I didn't see love between my mom and Albert, and I felt rejected by Albert and abandoned by my dad. Furthermore, my face was covered with pimples, and I could never get my hair to behave. This inspired disgust for my own body.

One day I had spent most of the afternoon working on my hair, trying to make it look decent. I had shampooed it, put it in curlers, and spent time under the hair dryer waiting for it to dry. Then I had brushed it, teased it, yelled at it, and despaired of ever being able to show my face in public again. Finally, I achieved a hairdo that I felt might possibly be presentable. I determined to forget my hair and see what was in the works for supper.

In the kitchen, Mom was running the mixer, signaling a possible cake in the making. When I drew close to see what she was doing, she turned and looked at me and said, "Veronica, why don't you do something with your hair, for heaven's sake?"

My world crashed into splinters at my feet. It didn't matter how hard I tried; I would never measure up.

My life had begun to feel like a deep pit, empty of meaning. What was the point, anyway? The only thing that kept me going was the sure knowledge that God was there and He loved me, and I wanted to make adequate preparations for an eternity in heaven with Him.

Eventually, however, I even began to question that. One night, I sat on the small throw rug on the wooden floor of my room and silently wailed, "God, are You really there? Is there an eternity to prepare for? You've got to show me, because if You don't, I have had it with this life. I'm going to end it. The struggle is not worth it."

Immediately, I felt God's hand lift me out of that pit. I heard Him say in my spirit, "Yes, I'm here, and I'm real, and there is an eternity to prepare for. It really is worth it."

I got up and went to bed, satisfied that there really was someone who loved me.

But even though from that point on I experienced a bedrock certainty of God's love for me in my spirit, I still didn't feel loved emotionally. Perhaps a better way to express it would be to say that I didn't know why anyone would love me, because I believed I fell so far short of anything worthwhile. I could trust that *God* loved me simply because that was His character. He *is* love, so He gives love to everyone, regardless of his or her worthiness. But I knew people were different for the most part. You had to meet expectations to be loved by people. Even when I did get feedback that told me I was loved, I couldn't accept it because I was watching so intently for rejection.

My childhood was a good one for the most part. I had plenty to eat, clothes to wear, a comfortable home to live in, a mother who took good care of me, and a stepfather who worked hard to provide for our family. I had lots of time to play. However, there were elements that added layers to my feelings of rejection.

For one thing, I was hardly ever disciplined. My mother felt bad about the effect of her divorce and remarriage on Don and me. Attempting to make up for that, she tried to sympathize with my needs. That translated into a reluctance to discipline me in any way. For example, I would bring home a pile of books from school every day. To get out of washing the supper dishes, I pointed to a ton of homework until Gail finished washing them. Then suddenly my homework was done and I could spend the rest of the evening watching TV. Mom never seemed to catch on to that ploy, but Gail saw right through it. It was a long time before her resentment faded.

I was a compliant person, eager to please the people around me, even though I was better at covering up lack of work than doing what was necessary. Perhaps Mom's lack of discipline produced in me a sort of victim mentality—the idea that because I had been shortchanged in the father area, I couldn't be expected to do the hard work other people had to do.

The point is that young people feel loved when they have firm guidelines lovingly imposed on them. Mom didn't do me any favors by not making me accountable for my actions. Although consciously I was glad to get out of doing things I didn't want to do, her lack of discipline translated to me subconsciously as rejection: I felt she didn't care enough about me to make sure I stayed on the right path. And because of that lack of discipline, I had to learn how to function in society in the school of hard knocks. By that I mean that for the most part I had to have external motivation for accomplishing anything. I was able to get up and go to work every day because I wanted enough money to maintain a certain standard of living, for example. I was sixty-one before I seriously attempted advanced education because I was never motivated enough before then. I didn't know how to relate properly to other people, so I mostly stayed to myself and concentrated on tasks.

Mom did get some important lessons through to me, however. Once when I was upset that I couldn't seem to please a friend, Mom explained, "For every person there is in the world, there is a whole different set of expectations. Even if you can figure out exactly what people expect of you, you can never fulfill all those various expectations for everyone. However, God has written His expectations in a book, and if you make it your business to study His Word, you can learn how to live a life that will please Him. If you please the Creator of the universe, everything else will fall into place. And if you please Him, why should you worry about what other people think of you?"

I still believe that is true. However, I have finally begun to understand that loving God and putting Him first in my life does not mean I shouldn't care about people. In fact, it means exactly the opposite. If I truly love God, I will also love people, because He loves people.

I was ten when my father remarried. Our stepmother, Evelyn, was all about discipline. I couldn't get away with anything when Don and I visited them in Wisconsin for two weeks every summer. (Our little sister Gail was the daughter of Mom and Albert, so she didn't join us on these trips.) I hated Evelyn because she was not as understanding as my mother, and I felt rejected because she *did* lovingly discipline me. You see how conflicted I was in this area.

Although at the time I despised Evelyn's detached way of making me accountable for my actions, I learned a lot from her without knowing it. I suspect that my tendency to go directly to solution mode when confronted with a problem came from her. In spite of myself, I admired her calmness in the face of my dad's fiery temper. In fact, she was the very reason his temper finally cooled. She had very little imagination, so when Daddy lost his temper about something, she had to ask him to explain why he was angry. By the time he finally told her enough so she understood the situation, he was no longer angry. Even then, she couldn't see what made him so angry, and I think he finally began to see things through her more rational eyes.

In addition, her insistence that I help around the house taught me useful skills I wouldn't have learned any other way. It was a long time before I appreciated that.

When I met my future husband, Jerry, in 1964, he and I were a classic example of being from different planets: he was from Mars; I was from Venus. Even though we were both Christians, our approaches to life were vastly different. His feet were solidly rooted in the soil of duty. If someone expected him to do something, he did it, come hell or high water. His logic brooked no nonsense about failing to perform just because he didn't feel like it. After we were married, he assumed I was completely onboard with the way he viewed things simply because he was the head of our home; and he was always astonished, and usually angry, whenever I disagreed.

I, on the other hand, never did anything unless the Spirit led, and the Spirit seldom led me to do anything productive. Our marriage would have been a great partnership had we valued each other's differences and learned from them, as we have finally learned to do. But we spent thirty years cutting each other to the quick with sarcasm before a book on intimacy finally opened our eyes to what was happening and helped us begin the process of changing it. We were both extremely opinionated, frequently believing entirely opposite things, and we both thought the other person should change to our way of viewing things.

For example, because I looked at life differently than he did, Jerry had a hard time believing I was being truthful when I expressed my opinions. He thought I must be either terribly naïve or lying. Several times when we couldn't come to an understanding about an issue, we knelt by our bed and talked to God about it out loud together. Jerry knew I loved God sincerely and I wouldn't lie to Him. Therefore, if I told God the same thing I had just told him, he would have to believe I really meant it. That very fact went a long way toward reaching a solution. Unfortunately, we usually argued for several hours before using prayer, the one thing that really worked, as a last resort.

Jerry was convinced he operated on the basis of logic, but his actions told me otherwise. If a problem presented itself, his first reaction once we had solved it was to talk about what we could do so this would *never happen again*. For example, he noticed once that lights were on all over the house, even in rooms that were not being used. He declared that we must get used to turning off lights when we left a room. His tone of voice indicated to me that he thought I was the main culprit here. Certainly, he would never do such a terribly wasteful thing.

I started turning lights off religiously in an effort to prove that I was not at fault. It also seemed like I spent my life following him around and turning off the lights that he left on. This fed my resentment of his inconsistencies.

Once I left a light on in a room, and he commented, "I thought we were going to turn off the lights when we left a room."

I shot back, "I'm just following your fine example."

Fortunately, for our marriage, since we were both from broken homes, we made a pact when we got married to stay together and be happy, even if it killed us.

A few times, it almost did.

Once I was so distraught that I thought about how good it would feel to drive my car into a brick wall at 60 mph and have it all over with. I don't remember why I didn't follow through with that—maybe I was still afraid of what people would think of me if I did. Maybe I just didn't know of a brick wall that I could trust to be firm enough to kill me and not just cause more pain.

This picture of my marriage may seem untenably barren, but there were considerations besides our pact that kept us together. For one thing, I was not sure of my own emotions. I believed that Jerry loved me, and I didn't know if anyone else would ever be as faithful to me as he was. Also, I was convinced that God would eventually teach us to express love for each other the way we both needed. I was unwilling to call a halt to the marriage before God had all the time He needed to pull that off. One of my favorite songs at the time had a verse that expressed this mentality: "Kiss me each morning for a million years. Hold me each evening by your side. Tell me you love me for a million years. Then if it don't work out, if it don't work out, Then you can tell me goodbye."[5]

---

5   Lyrics to "Then You Can Tell Me Goodbye" by John D. Loudermill, accessed August 2, 2012. http://www.oldielyrics.com/lyrics/the_casinos/then_you_can_tell_me_goodbye.html.

Besides that, I was just plain lazy. One day I actually considered divorce, but I took a good look at all the stuff in our garage, not to mention the house, and the prospect of dividing it all up equitably just made me tired. My attitude of not having to do the hard work others had to do finally stood me in good stead and helped save my marriage.

Although my head knew that Jerry loved me, I didn't feel it in my heart for many years. In fact, I felt rejected by him most of the time. He really tried to show his love for me by being faithful to our marriage, by providing a good living for our family, and by doing romantic things like remembering special occasions and buying me nice gifts. For example, one year he bought me an oak roll-top desk for my birthday—an item I had been drooling over for some time. One of my favorite gifts from him was a three-hole punch—this communicated the message that he cherished my practical bent and was willing to provide me with the tools I needed to do the things I loved. On the other hand, whenever I wanted to have a conversation with him, he had an annoying habit of checking his watch, sending me the message that he thought everything else in his life was more important than spending time talking with me. The pattern of perceiving only rejection had been set in motion long ago, and I gave far more weight to the small annoying things he did than to the many loving things. I did not know how to see the love, set aside my harsh judgments of his shortcomings, and let the rejection messages go.

I projected this same rejection to all the other people in my life. In an effort to protect myself from the dreaded rejection, I was always on the lookout for it, and I frequently picked it up even when it didn't exist. My defense became to do everything right so nobody would have grounds for rejecting me. But perfection has never inspired love. In fact, if you were perfect, people would probably hate you as they hated Jesus. But I wasn't perfect (perhaps you've already picked up on that), and the very fact that I was depending on my perfect performance to be accepted meant that when I did not succeed, I saw myself as being rejected—even if nobody else rejected me for that reason.

I think in my quest to do all things perfectly I projected a picture to the world of having it all together. I never asked for help. I didn't want to impose on others unless it was absolutely necessary. I didn't believe anyone would come to my aid unless I was dying or something. This did not encourage close relationships.

Through the years, God gradually began opening my eyes to my need for intimate connections with people. The summer of 2004, when I was fifty-eight, Jerry and I went to a picnic with other members of our church. Everyone was engaged in conversations except me. I kept trying to join the conversations, but it seemed like I didn't fit in anywhere. I had considered retiring later that year, but I hesitated because I knew how hard it was for me to be self-motivated about anything. I could make myself go to work because there was a paycheck to anticipate, but I didn't know if there was anything I wanted to do enough to make me do it without that monetary incentive. After that picnic, I felt a clear impression in my spirit that after I retired, God would be helping me work on relationships. The process began even before I retired at the end of November, when I was asked to direct the Christmas outreach program of our church. That led to becoming director of the Mercy Ministry, which involved providing food and groceries for those in need. In 2007, I began a two-year biblical counseling course that rocked my world and gave God a platform for dealing with many of my issues.

In 2009, my sixty-third year, God made it clear to me exactly what happened in my heart way back when I was feeling rejection and abandonment from Albert and my father. In the deep place of my childish heart, I had built a wall around it to keep people at a distance, so I would never again feel that rejection and abandonment. I relegated everybody in the world to the category of people-who-would-hurt-me-if-they-ever-got-the-chance. Since I would never do such a terrible thing, I figured I was eligible to sit in the seat of God and pass judgment on everyone else. However, there is a spiritual law that says if you judge others, you must also judge yourself.[6] And since indwelling sin[7] was

---

6   See Romans 2:1.
7   See Romans 7:17. The Bible teaches that indwelling sin is a force within each of us

always there magnifying every bad thing I felt about myself, I ended up condemning myself. So on one hand, I thought I was good enough to judge other people, but on the other hand, I hated myself at least as much as I hated everyone else. I was tearing myself apart. This went on for nearly sixty years.

During the thirty years I worked as a rural-route mail carrier with the Postal Service, my life mostly focused on tasks rather than relationships. I did have friends, but I didn't spend much time with them. I had a husband and two children, but my relationships with them consisted mostly of the tasks involved in caring for a house and family rather than taking the time to enjoy them. I was involved in my church, but again, I was mostly performing tasks rather than enjoying relationships.

For the five years prior to this revelation in 2009, God had been gently and gradually shepherding me away from my task-orientation and toward relationships. Tasks were easy—cut and dried, no messy emotions to deal with, no misunderstandings. Just do the work and feel the satisfaction of a job well done. However, more and more, I felt bored with tasks and I felt an increasing need to interact with people. But there was a wall between me and other people that kept me from satisfying connections with them. It felt like that wall was ten feet high, three feet wide, and made of impenetrable concrete. It didn't seem that people wanted to hang out with me, and if they ever did, I could never think of anything to say or do to encourage a connection.

One day I wasn't even thinking about that issue when God brought to my mind the holographic images of a room full of Civil War-era people dancing, which I had seen at the Disneyland haunted house. He showed me that the wall between other people and me was not made of concrete after all. Rather, it was more like a holographic image. All I had to do to get rid of it was turn off the projection machine. It was so simple that it was breathtaking. My heart exploded with joy at the

---

that endlessly goads us to do precisely the opposite of anything God would have us do. One of its functions is to bring condemnation of self and others in our minds. See Revelation 12:10, where Satan, and by extension indwelling sin, is called the accuser of the brethren.

thought that relationships could be within my grasp. Quickly a cloud gathered, however.

"But there's a problem, Lord," I said. "How do I turn off that machine?"

"Just give up your perceived right to judge other people," came the answer deep in my spirit. *How easy was that?* For years, God had been pointing out Scriptures that highlighted His hatred of the way people passed judgment on others. That understanding brought me to a critical point of conviction and surrender in that moment.

"Yes!" I cried. "I give it up right now!"

In subsequent months, God helped me recognize the extent of my habit of judging people. It was almost never a matter of confronting someone's misdeeds. It was more a heart attitude that was never expressed in words to the person being judged. For example, once I saw a man riding a bicycle without a helmet, and my reaction was, "Well, he probably doesn't have any brains to protect." Bingo! The Lord pointed out my attitude of judgment. It was toxic to all my relationships, even if the person I was silently judging never knew what I was thinking.

With the holographic projector turned off, the wall between other people and me crumbled and I began to learn how to build relationships. In the fall of 2009, I began taking classes at Front Range Community College in Fort Collins, Colorado, working slowly toward a master's degree in counseling at the rate of one class per semester. My first class was Psychology 101.

God did some amazing things in my heart during that semester. For one thing, He opened my eyes so I could see the gold in my teacher and my classmates. I was the oldest student in the class, and this was my first formal school experience in thirty-five years. I had to scramble to learn modern classroom procedures, and my brain felt rusty. My classmates responded to our teacher's questions with lightning speed. While I was still trying to figure out what in the heck his question was asking, they already had ten answers ready. I was blown away with their quick minds. In addition, each of them had a uniquely engaging personality.

I marveled at God's genius in creating each person so wonderfully different, and I rejoiced that He allowed me the privilege of knowing them for a short time.

Then there was our subject matter itself. We spent time examining various aspects of the human body, such as the eyes, the ears, and the digestive and nervous systems. My brain was whirling at 100 mph, 24/7. I could barely sleep because of the enormity of these revelations. I loved my iPhone, but next to the human body, it was a piece of junk.

God was also helping me reconnect with my emotions after decades of refusing to feel them in favor of taking care of all my tasks. In addition to helping me connect with people, the dismantling of my wall had precipitated an onslaught of unaccustomed sentiments. It was a veritable hurricane of amazing revelations that fueled a whirlpool of emotions.

Even after the semester ended, I could not rest because I was so amazed by all I had learned. Finally, I asked God why I couldn't let these things go and get some sleep. He answered, giving me this understanding in my spirit: "It's good that you see the gold in other people and that you appreciate the amazing intricacy of creation. But you shouldn't *worship* these things. You should only worship Me."

That answered a question that had been on the back burner of my mind for a long time—what exactly is worship? Somehow, singing a few songs and listening to a sermon on Sunday morning never seemed to adequately define worship for me, even though it was called a worship service. But this cast a whole new light on the subject. Yes, I thought, having your entire being wrapped up in something—I can see how that would be worship.

This experience helped me appreciate the beauty in people while not leaning on them for my sustenance and self-esteem. But it was not until I faced the potentially life-threatening prospect of breast cancer that I learned yet another dimension of personal relationships, and it all began to come together for me.

Chapter 3

The Truth: When He Has Tested Me, I Will Come Forth as Gold

After my diagnosis in the summer of 2011, the next practical step was stopping the hormone therapy I had been on for more than twenty years. In my forties, my dormant PMS had returned with a vengeance after a hiatus of several years. My doctor recommended estrogen and progesterone to mitigate the symptoms. Through the years, we had tweaked the dosage until now I was humming along with nary a glitch—except, of course, for the cancer. Cancer loves estrogen, so now that we knew cancer was there, we needed to stop feeding it. Unfortunately, I didn't know how that would affect me. I had tried weaning myself off the estrogen before, but the hot flashes drove me back to it.

I was actually more afraid of hot flashes that might result from the lack of estrogen in my system than I was of the cancer. And yet I determined to approach that move with equanimity. I was sixty-five, for Pete's sake. I should be done with hot flashes. Although I did subsequently have hot flashes, they were never severe, and I found that accepting them and rolling with their challenge robbed them of their teeth.

On June 1, 2011, almost two months before my diagnosis, I had started a new list of Bible verses to memorize. Every morning I worked on a list of about twenty-five new verses, as well as systematically reviewing some of the six hundred verses I had memorized in the last fifteen years. I memorize Scripture because it feeds my spirit just as food nourishes my physical body. I want to know God. I want Him to have a broad spectrum of His Word available in me so He can remind me of it when I need a course correction. This body of Scripture is a solid foundation, like a faithful sheepdog that shepherds me onto the right path.

One of my favorite verses on the new list was Job 23:10 (NIV): "But he knows the way that I take; when he has tested me I will come forth as gold." The price of gold that summer was $1,616 an ounce. At approximately 140 pounds, I figured I should be worth $1,034,240 when this was done! But of course, God's worth far exceeds gold, so I looked forward to having the Midas touch in the spirit at the end of this journey.

One of the first things I did after my diagnosis was set up a blog to keep family and friends informed of my progress.[8] I shared not only the facts about my cancer journey but also the deep, life-changing insights God was giving me. I was astonished when people responded to my blog entries. People frequently thanked me for keeping them updated in this way. Sometimes they commented on how inspiring my story was to them. My neighbor lady always looked forward to the next installment of what she affectionately called my "soap opera." The simple fact that people were actually reading my blog entries communicated love to me, and their positive responses affirmed that my life might actually have some kind of value to others.

The next thing I thought about upon receiving the cancer diagnosis was a book I had heard about several months earlier. At a dinner gathering, some friends had expressed intrigue about the story of a young woman who decided against conventional cancer treatments in favor of a holistic approach. I thought at the time that if I ever did get cancer, which I never would, of course, I would do the same thing.

---

8   The two websites I heard about were mylifeline.org and caringbridge.org. I chose mylifeline.org.

Upon receiving my diagnosis, I immediately contacted my friends, found out the title of the book—*You Did What?* by Hollie and Patrick Quinn—and ordered it.[9]

Hollie had been diagnosed with stage two aggressive breast cancer in her thirty-eighth week of pregnancy. Her doctor told her she must have surgery immediately, followed by chemo, radiation, and hormone therapy, or she would die. *Period.* After the birth of her child, she did have the surgery. But then she and her husband researched the conventional cancer treatments and found they actually did very little to free a person from the threat of cancer, not to mention extend patients' lives. Instead, they stripped the immune system of the ability to do its job of searching out and destroying cancer cells before they became a problem. There also appeared to be a strong correlation between these treatments and cancer that recurred several years down the road in other, less accessible parts of the body, such as the brain or major organs.

Hollie and her husband decided to forgo the conventional cancer treatments and instead use botanical supplements to strengthen her immune system. Eleven years later, she has never been more robustly healthy, having had no reoccurrence of cancer.

After reading the book myself, I was even more convinced that the nonconventional approach was the best one. But of course, that was not the end of the story. There were other considerations, such as the cost of those supplements. They were not cheap, and no insurance would cover them. Also, my husband had a different view of things. Supplements had never worked for him so he believed that conventional medicine was the way to go. He was not willing to place my life in the hands of a treatment protocol that had not been through the same rigorous testing of conventional medicines.

Never mind that there were very good reasons why that testing had not taken place. Mainly it had to do with economic incentive. Natural substances could not be patented and therefore could not become the exclusive property of any given company. Therefore, no one was about

---

9   Hollie and Patrick Quinn. *You Did What? Saying "No" to Conventional Cancer Treatment.* Cobblestone Publishing, LLC, 2010.

to spend millions of dollars on the testing that was needed to comply with FDA standards. Therefore, substances that had been used for thousands of years to successfully treat many physical conditions and to strengthen the immune system were being effectively denied to citizens of the richest, most medically advanced country in the world. These people were dying from diseases that in many cases could be cured, but since the cures were not endorsed by the medical community and were not covered by insurance, people did not know about them, did not trust them, or could not afford them. Or all of the above.

A series of conversations ensued between Jerry and me concerning my treatment path. In the beginning of this process, I told Jerry that I did not want to do anything that he wasn't completely in agreement with. I did not want to order expensive supplements, only to have him roll his eyes and resent the money we were spending on them. A couple days later, he came to me and said, "I want you to know that I will fully support whatever decision you make."

This was a first in our forty-six-year marriage. Jerry usually had a pretty good idea of what he wanted, and I usually didn't, so it was easy for me to accommodate myself to his decisions, support him, and go along for the ride. I liked supporting him and my children in their endeavors. Certainly, I expressed strong opinions on things numerous times through the years, but I was usually happy to let him make the final decision. I was glad I wasn't in the position of having to be the final decision maker.

This statement suddenly put me in a position of responsibility. He trusted me to make a wise decision concerning my health and our finances. My decision would not only affect me but him, as well as our standard of living. If I suffered with conventional treatments, he might have to stand by, unable to help me feel better. If I tried the natural supplements instead and they didn't do the trick, he might have to watch me die and try to figure out how to live without me. It was time to grow up and think deeply about this.

When I told our daughter, Jen, about my diagnosis, she felt gut-punched. "How do *you* feel about it?" she asked when she recovered her voice.

I said something like, "I'm actually stoked about it. I need structure, and I didn't have any this summer. I was floating, and I don't like floating. This is something I can get my teeth into. Suddenly I know what I have to do."

"Mom," she said, exasperated, "you can take a class or something if you need structure. You don't have to get cancer!"

We discussed the reasons why we both hated the idea of cancer. "I just don't want to die," she said.

"Really?" I was surprised. "I don't have a problem with death. In fact, let me go see my new house in heaven! I just want to avoid the pain of the disease and the treatments. Don't you think about the pain?"

"No," she said as she shook her head. "The prospect of pain doesn't bother me that much. I just want to go on living."

Jerry's willingness to abide by my final decision did not mean he did not let me know his thoughts. At one point, he and I had each become entrenched in our opposing thoughts about this subject, and we needed help talking to each other about it.

Our son, Steve, and his wife, Aleisha, came over one evening to facilitate a discussion concerning treatment options after surgery. Steve is a gifted facilitator and wonderfully able to keep the discussion on point. Aleisha offered a softer side, understanding our feelings. Together, they were able to encourage us to listen to each other's hearts and take each other's concerns into account. That discussion was a turning point for my husband and me, making it possible for us to be on the same page.

Steve opened the discussion. "So, what are the issues we are dealing with here?"

I didn't feel there *was* an issue, so I waited for Jerry to respond. He sat back in his recliner and crossed his legs. "I guess the main issue is Veronica's treatment path once she has the mastectomy. If chemo or radiation is recommended, that's the route I'd want her to take, but she doesn't like that idea."

That inspired a response and I jumped in. "My body is so fine-tuned and reacts so strongly to meds that I shudder to think what that stuff would do to me. I can't even take over-the-counter pain meds because they give me hives." (The hormone therapy I had taken for twenty years predated my allergy to over-the-counter pain meds. Back then I just did what the doctor said and didn't worry about it. That had changed.)

"Really?" Steve was astonished. "That's scary. What would you want to do instead of chemo and radiation?"

"I think it makes a lot more sense to take supplements that strengthen the body's immune system so it can defend itself like it was designed to do. That's what I'd like to do."

"That makes sense to me," Aleisha offered from her seat beside Steve on the couch. "I know my body strongly objects to some things too. How do you feel about that, Dad?"

"I don't mind the supplements, but I do object to going bankrupt because of them," Jerry declared, his voice rising. "That stuff is expensive, and no insurance is going to help us with it."

"What about that, Mom?" Steve asked. "Do you have any idea how you could pay for the supplements?"

I sat forward in my recliner, leaning into the argument. "We're getting a loan payment every month that we've been putting into a savings account. We haven't designated it for anything yet, so I think we could say it's available for that. I'd like to see if the clinic in Oregon could design a protocol that we could pay for with that."

Jerry sighed. "I'm very suspicious of that kind of thing. I'm afraid they'll try to convince you that you need to buy everything they recommend or you'll get cancer again."

I was starting to get upset. "I don't intend to spend all our money on supplements, and if they can't work within our budget, I'll just say no. I don't see anything wrong with at least talking with them to see what they can do for us. You can be on the phone call with me. You can hang up the phone if I get carried away."

"That sounds reasonable to me," Steve said. "What do you think, Dad?"

"Well, maybe that would be a good way to do it," Jerry agreed.

After more discussion, we agreed to table the matter until we learned the pathology report and the oncologist's recommendation and we could talk to Jonathon at the Oregon clinic about working within our budget on the supplements.

Chapter 4

Weeding the Garden: God Fights for Me

I also had an ongoing conversation with the Lord. There were so many things I did not know about the future of my cancer journey. I didn't know if the surgery would reveal that the tumor was contained or if it had metastasized (spread to other parts of my body). I didn't know what treatment the oncologist would recommend after surgery or what the odds would be if I did or did not choose to follow that recommendation. Finally, overwhelmed by all the possibilities and choices, I laid it all at God's feet and surrendered to His plan, whatever it might be.

"Father," I said, "I don't know which way to go here. Only You know what will result from any decision I might make. And only You know the best possible course of action for me. Please guide Jerry and me in our decision-making process so we will be in complete agreement. Whatever You want is okay with me—whether it's instant healing, surgery, chemo with whatever comes with it, years of agony as I fight cancer, or death. I only want Your guidance and presence every step of the way. I know that whatever You want for me will be the best possible thing, the path of ultimate safety, and You will give me strength for it."

It seemed to take forever to schedule appointments with the surgeon and the plastic surgeon, since their schedules were hard to mesh, and then another forever to schedule the surgery, for the same reason. I had heard of other cases, like Hollie's in the book, where surgery was scheduled quickly. I suppose there was not so much urgency in my case because my tumor was so small and apparently not aggressive. I didn't mind that it took so long, because I really wanted to attend our church's leadership retreat in mid-August, as well as another retreat in September. I was elated when surgery was scheduled for September 12, the Monday after that September retreat. Those retreats brought me a lot of peace as I anticipated surgery.

Although there was never any fear of cancer, there was plenty of anxiety concerning my treatment path following surgery. This anxiety was hardly ever conscious. It stayed beneath the radar, with me feeling just fine consciously until it popped out in the form of hives, which began to appear more frequently and severely. Usually one or two Claritin tablets a day took care of it, but I felt sure that anxiety was at its root a spiritual problem, and I did everything I knew to get my mind off the myriad of cancer treatment options and rest in God's ability to show me the right path.

For example, one day Jerry and I took a bike ride on the extensive bike paths in our town. That morning, I had had a few itchy hives spots—a sure sign of anxiety. As I rode my bike, I intentionally began to think about all the things I could be thankful for, and there were plenty: the cool cloud cover; the fact that the Lord was holding back the rain as we wound our way home; the infinite variety of trees and vegetation along the path; the fragrance of freshly mown grass; the strength God gave me for the ride, even though I had been feeling weak that morning for some reason; and lots more. As I rode, I gave thanks to God for all these things, and I kept that up all day whenever I thought of something else to be thankful for. There were no hives that evening.

Another sure sign of underground anxiety was what I called my "fuzzy-brain syndrome." I started forgetting things and it became difficult to function as crisply as I had before. It seemed to me that this was another symptom of anxiety rather than a physical symptom, since I was not on any drugs and had not experienced any sickness due to the cancer. It was an indication to me that there was still some disconnect between what I believed about God being fully in control and how I really felt about things. There was still work to be done in letting God's truth saturate my innermost being.

I wondered at times if my lack of conscious fear was healthy. Surely, if I had a realistic handle on things, I would be afraid of cancer. And yet I was doing the best I knew to live out what I knew to be true: that I could be thankful for all things[10] because God was in control and if I loved Him, He would work everything out for my good and His glory.[11] There was a very real battle being waged in my mind. Every moment of every day, I had a choice to either be depressed and anxious about all the things that could possibly go wrong or to be thankful that God was in control. My conscious choice was always to be thankful and trust God to work things out, but I also believed that hives and fuzzy-brain syndrome were symptoms of subconscious anxiety. I did not know how to treat that, but I was sure God would address that issue in due time.

The decision concerning my treatment path began with several options regarding the surgery itself. I could have a lumpectomy, which was a viable option since my tumor appeared to be very small. The surgeon would simply remove the tumor and a little surrounding tissue. There would be no reconstruction with that, and that breast would forever be a different shape than the other one. In addition, radiation would be recommended, since there would be a 25 percent chance that cancer cells would still be present after that surgery.

Or I could have a mastectomy, removing the entire breast. I am still not clear about all the mastectomy options—there were several—but I chose the one that was supposed to do a very good job of reconstruction while requiring only six weeks to recover, as opposed to three months of recovery for the surgery that included a tummy tuck. When I briefly thought longingly of the tummy tuck option, Jerry wisely pointed out that three months of recovery was not something either of us really wanted. The surgery that only took six weeks of recovery

---

10   Ephesians 5:20.
11   Romans 8:28.

would accomplish our goal of a great reconstruction, and I could learn a little self-discipline in my eating habits to deal with the excess tummy fat. With the mastectomy, there would be only a 2 percent chance that cancer cells remained, so there would be no radiation after that. We decided to go with the six-week-recovery mastectomy.

In her book, Hollie stated that she would have skipped surgery had she known at the start what she found out later about the power of good nutritional supplements. But from my first conversation with my doctor, surgery seemed to be a foregone conclusion. Jerry and our kids all felt strongly that we needed to get the tumor out of there, and after some thought and prayer, I agreed.

Besides the surgery options, I discovered there were lots of ways other than conventional treatments that seemed to have been effective in curing people of cancer. Most of them were expensive, not covered by insurance, and labor intensive. And who could know if they would work for me? I began to read a book that told about many of these treatment options. For example, there was the Hoxsey therapy, a completely herbal treatment available in Tijuana; Essiac herbal tea available online, but I didn't know how pure it would be; and the Gerson method that included five coffee enemas a day, thirteen fresh juices a day, and a very strict diet of no salt, no sugar, little fat or meat, and nutritional supplementation.[12] I felt I needed to know about all the available options, but I couldn't see how any of them would be practical for me.

Soon my brain was on overload from thinking about all these options, and fuzzy-brain syndrome kicked in with a vengeance. Then one day God gave me an object lesson about how to deal with all the options. I recorded it in my 8/22/11 blog entry.

> I have to tell you about our little flower garden in front
> of our house. It hasn't had much attention at all this
> summer, what with Jerry's knee surgery in May and

---

12   Pierce, Tanya Harter. *Outsmart Your Cancer: Alternative Non-Toxic Treatments That Work* Stateline. Nevada: Thoughtworks Publishing 2004.

now this cancer diagnosis. This afternoon, I needed to do some reading and the house was frigid from the AC. Even the back deck was cool because it was in the shade. I decided to sit in one of the little chairs on our front patio, facing the street, but even that was in the shade and cool at that time of the day. So I put the chair on the grass where there was still sunlight, but since I didn't want to face the sun, I turned my chair toward the house and the flower garden instead, with my back to the sun. I got comfortable and started to read.

Soon I looked up and saw a weed growing in the garden. *I should just pull it out of there,* I thought. Then I noticed all the long grasses that were growing among the flowers in that area, and I started pulling those out by the roots, one by one. Presently I noticed the same grasses in other areas of the garden and began pulling them. Finally, I saw that the daisies had pretty much died off and were just a bunch of ugly deadheads, and I felt the need to cut them back. It wasn't long before I had several large mounds of weeds and deadheads around the edge of the garden, and the garden was looking really great. I could feel the flower plants breathing deeply and giving thanks that the weeds no longer strangled them.

The spiritual lesson that came to mind in all this was God's gentle prodding in motivating me to do a task that needed to be done. First getting me outside, then into the sun but facing away from the sun and toward the house and the garden, then shining a spotlight on that one big weed. Once He had my attention, He was able to communicate the need to pull all those weeds.

My research into cancer treatments is like that, I guess. Little by little, doing what I can, trusting that God will open doors, following leads, and starting to put the pieces together into a big picture. Fortunately, I do not feel the need to rush into a decision here. I believe at the right time I will know exactly what to do and it will be the right thing.[13]

I asked for help from my Mercy Ministry team at church because I was having trouble processing all the details of the ministry. One lady took over the financial assistance portion of the ministry, and my Food Pantry director assumed my duties as overall director until I could return to my full strength. They were happy to do this—not one of them ever resented the extra work, and they were always checking to see if I was okay.

My other friends at church were also unfailingly gentle and solicitous toward me. I began to believe that if I needed them to help in any way, they would gladly do it.

Another problem of researching all the treatment options was that I became focused on cancer, as much as I was trying not to. God gave me another object lesson about that.

One day we took our daughter, Jen, and her two daughters, Bailey and Cadie, ages thirteen and eleven, to Water World for the day. The weather was perfect—warm, with clouds gathering in the afternoon to keep us from roasting. My mindset lately had been tunnel vision focused on education regarding cancer and treatment options. Early in the day at Water World, the Lord said to me, "You need to forget about cancer for a while and have some fun." Well, you should know I've never been much good at having fun, on my best day. That's one reason God gave

---

13   Arnold, Veronica. August 2, 2011 blog entry, http://www.mylifeline.org/page. cfm?page=getstarted. To access my blog, please e-mail me at grangle@q.com and I will send you an invitation. The blog provides all the details of my cancer journey, from the diagnosis to my final recovery. There is background in this book that does not appear in the blog, and there are daily details in the blog that did not seem to add to the narrative of this particular story.

me Jerry, who frequently yanks me out of my comfortable task-oriented rut, kicking and screaming, and insists that I enjoy myself. Usually I don't even hear the music they play over loud speakers in public places. But suddenly I was hearing the music, feeling the beat, and doing a funky little dance while we walked along the pathways. I'm sure Jen was thinking, *Who are you, and what have you done with my mom?* I forgot about cancer, and we all had a good time.

Of course, the lesson here was that *I* was not cancer. I didn't even like to say that I *had* cancer but that I had been *diagnosed* with cancer. Even then, cancer insinuated itself as my identity, with all the information I had to gather and all the people I needed to talk to. I asked my blog readers to pray that I would spend the necessary time being still in God's presence and worshipping Him so that I would always remember I am His child, He lives in me, and *that's* who I am. And that I would continue to be involved at church and reach out to others as a good ongoing reminder that I was not the only one going through a challenging situation. It was a continual battle between resting in God's truth and believing the lies of indwelling sin.

I began attending a breast cancer support group once a month. It was facilitated by an oncologist social worker who was knowledgeable about all aspects of the cancer journey. She was also a very compassionate person, expressing great appreciation for the courage of every breast cancer patient who attended.

I saw this compassion in everyone I encountered in the medical community as I prepared for surgery, as well as everyone who learned I was dealing with cancer. My old view of people as those-who-would-hurt-me-if-they-got-the-chance was being radically challenged.

My husband's attitude changed as well. Suddenly, he was faced with the possibility that I might not be around forever, and he became more thoughtful and kind than ever before. When I had trouble getting things done because my brain was fuzzy and slow to function, he pitched in and helped. A deeper awareness of each other kicked in to help him know what I needed. Up to this time, neither of us had needed the help of the other on this level, although his recent knee replacement was good training for this. Like many married couples, we had each taken care of our separate responsibilities, helping each other occasionally, but mostly living somewhat separate lives. It felt wonderful to experience his thoughtfulness and tender care now that I needed it.

Our adult children and their families also stepped up to the relationship plate. Jen and Steve were both eager to talk whenever I called them. They took the initiative and planned outings with us. This touched me deeply.

Jerry's ninety-seven-year-old mother, Gram Zook, called me frequently to make sure I was feeling okay, even though I never had any pain or sickness as a result of the cancer. The only real problem was the stress of figuring out my treatment path. Whenever I sent her a paper copy of a blog entry (she didn't have access to the Internet), she would always call to discuss it with me. She prayed fervently for me all the time. Even though her eyesight and hearing were fading, she never complained about her own problems. Her only concern was for me.

During that fall, I attended four retreats—one with the leadership of our church, one with the Mercy Ministry, one with the women of our church, and one with a group of women from my biblical counseling course. At each one, I was treated with tenderness and affection.

In addition, God used those opportunities when I was still to communicate awesome truths about His love for me. Here is a particularly vivid picture He brought to my mind as I quieted myself and listened to Him at one of those retreats.

> Jesus and I are at the altar as bride and groom. I gaze on Him with delight—He is the most deliriously handsome, strong, awesome bridegroom I could ever imagine. He looks at me tenderly and holds out to me His wedding gift. I know what it is—His eternal, unconditional, unchanging love—but I hesitate to receive it. Why is there any hesitation? I desperately want this gift. I need

it just to keep on breathing. Why the hesitation? What lie holds me back?

There are actually two lies. One lie says I am so unworthy of His love. How can I have the temerity to even think about reaching out and taking it when I am such a worm? But the truth is He created me from the beginning as a precious and perfect jewel. It is true that I have been dipped in the mud, but His blood has wiped me clean so I can shine again in His light. *He* has *made* me worthy to receive the gift.

The other lie says this is not socially acceptable. It's just not the way weddings are done. The gift must be given at another time, in another place. This love is a private matter and it is in severely bad taste to receive it right in front of all the wedding guests. But the truth is that He is the wedding master and any time, place, and way He wants to give the gift is appropriate and beautiful.

So I accept the truth of who He says I am, reckon myself dead to all the lies,[14] and with joy receive that delightful gift of His love. I step into His arms, we turn to face the guests, and together we go forth as beloved bride and triumphant groom.

---

14 This is a reference to Romans 6:11, which tells us to believe the truth that we are dead to sin—we no longer have to be a slave to it—and instead alive only to God.

Chapter 5

God Is with Me: No Need to Fear

I had my mastectomy in September. It seems like it should have been a big deal, since it was pretty much the centerpiece of my cancer treatment, but once the decision was made, I was happy to have it over with. Of course, I was unconscious during the surgery, and for several days after surgery I was on pain pills and Valium so there was no pain and I was in a pleasant fog. Therefore, the surgery itself seemed somewhat anticlimactic.

The only complication was when I passed out in the bathroom the night after the surgery, resulting in a code blue and needing a nurse whenever I got out of bed for the rest of my hospital stay. I joked that I only did that so I could be the center of attention. Of course, I didn't do it on purpose, but it did make me the center of attention!

For that thirty-hour stay, I drank gallons of water and made numerous trips to the bathroom to get rid of it. And every time I needed a water bottle refill or a trip to the bathroom, I had to summon a nurse. I began to feel like I must be the only patient on the floor because I never had to wait more than sixty seconds for someone to respond to my call. I was extremely impressed with the care I received at Poudre Valley Hospital.

There were six weeks of recovery at home. During that time, I was under doctor's orders to avoid exercise, except for an easy routine of left arm, shoulder, and neck exercises they gave me to keep things loose on that side as I healed. I took a narcotic pain medication for a few days and Valium for ten days.

Jerry spent half his life refilling my water bottle during that time, since I didn't have the strength in my hands to get the top off. He slept in his recliner in the living room so I could have the entire bed to myself. I just about needed it all too, by the time I piled pillows on my left side to keep my arm elevated and kept a TV tray by the bed on my right side to keep my water bottle handy throughout the night. I learned later that he was careful to wear his outfits several days in a row rather than using clean clothes every day, to cut down on the amount of laundry and ironing that had to be done. In my pain pill/Valium fog, I did vaguely notice a small pile of his clothes on the living room couch, but I didn't have the energy to even be curious about it.

I took a lot of naps during those days and had a lot of dreams. Frequently, I dreamed that I was reaching over to get my water bottle and bringing it over to get a drink, but then I realized no water was going into my mouth. When I woke up, I had a real drink of water. It was a fascinating blend of dreams and reality.

Jerry worked on earning his "master chef" certificate. One day, for example, he wanted to make tomato soup for us for lunch. While he opened the can and poured the soup into a bowl, I sat at the dining room table and coached him. "Don't forget to pour in a soup can full of milk and stir it with a wire whisk. That's in the utensil holder by the stove."

He found the utensil holder, and then he finally found something that looked like a wire whisk. "This?" he asked.

"Yep. Good job!"

After he stirred the soup adequately, I continued. "Get one of the medium-size plates in the cupboard and put the bowl on it. That way, you'll be able to get the bowl out of the microwave without burning your fingers. Then another medium-size plate on top of the bowl will keep the soup from spattering all over the microwave."

Once the soup was in the microwave, he asked, "How long do I set the oven for?"

"Set it for five minutes on medium heat."

"What? What is medium heat?"

"Whenever you heat something in the microwave," I explained, "the automatic heat setting is high unless you change it. Sometimes you need a lower heat setting so food will warm up more evenly. To do that, punch in 5 0 0 for the time, then the 'power level' button and 5 for the heat setting."

"Why not just set it for three minutes on high?" he asked. "Then it would be done quicker."

"It would also boil over and the milk would curdle," I explained.

Having set the oven properly, he wondered what to do next.

"I'd like a piece of bread to break up into my soup," I suggested. "The bread is in the garage refrigerator."

He brought in the bread, found crackers in the cupboard for himself, and cut some cheese to have on the side.

I loved it that he was listening to my directions, following them, and even discussing the reasons for them. When he brought the perfectly heated soup to the table, I rewarded him with a warm smile and a hug. "Very nice," I said. "We'll make a master chef out of you yet."

In subsequent lessons, he learned where the plastic storage containers were in the kitchen and began to get a feel for which size to use for which leftovers. I loved the companionship of doing those things with him. He was an absolute prince about making sure he was available when I needed him. He has always been good about doing little things to rescue me, but during this time, he became my hero in a whole new way.

The pathology report at my next oncology appointment was fabulous: the margins of the tumor were clear of cancer cells, and there were no cancer cells in my lymph nodes. My oncologist didn't recommend chemo *or* radiation, and I opted out of the hormone therapy she suggested because of the possible threat of bone loss. That therapy would have removed estrogen from my system. Although that would be good for preventing future cancers, it would also deny my bones the benefit of estrogen. Instead of hormone therapy, I ordered supplements from the Oregon clinic designed for me based on my blood work. Jonathon had prescribed a protocol of supplements that nicely fit into our budget.

Although I was not allowed to lift things or do much of anything with my arms for six weeks after my surgery, there were things that had to be done around the house. I still needed my fruit and veggie smoothies, for example. I had been drinking these smoothies for about three years as an easy way to get a great variety of fruit and veggies I would not ordinarily eat, and I felt they were even more important now. Twice during that time, people came over to help me make large batches to freeze. Once Jen and her daughters came over and helped me. I coached them about washing and chopping the veggies. I was very impressed with how helpful Bailey and Cadie were in that process, and the whole thing was a lot of fun. It reminded me of the big family holiday dinners we had when I was a child, when all the women and girls gathered in the kitchen after the meal to wash the dishes—fond memories of family camaraderie. This experience aided the process of beginning to give more weight to the loving memories of my childhood and diminish the rejection memories.

Once my friend, Marguerite, brought her juicer over, along with a big bag of beets with their greens, spinach, carrots, green beans, and apples. She proceeded to make several jars of her super-duper green juice and even vacuum-sealed them. The juice was quite tasty, actually. It was also extremely high in nutrients—apparently without the fiber, the juice is digested much more easily and delivered to the cells faster. This communicated love not only emotionally but also physically, as the juice helped me recover faster.

Marguerite also came over one day and helped me make three kinds of soup so our family could celebrate three October birthdays. That was such a lot of fun, making it possible for us to host our family celebration dinner.

Another friend, Kim, offered her assistance in any way I might need it. Since the lady who normally cleaned our house once a month was also laid up from surgery, I asked Kim if she would like to clean house for me. She was delighted. She said it was rare when people responded to such offers. She did a great job and we had some time to chat and catch up with one another. Although we live in the same town, we hadn't gotten together in several years.

I thought about how God must feel. He offers to help us in every situation of our lives. He is always available. Numerous times in the Bible, He tells us to ask for what we want and need and He will take care of it. In the book of Ephesians, He says we can't even imagine all the things He wants to do for us,[15] but how many of us actually take Him up on those promises and trust Him to keep them?

I mentioned in my blog that Abba (Father God) was so good to send me people with skin on. Someone asked what that meant and if I was entertaining people who had no skin. I replied, "We certainly do experience God's love directly from Him, but He also likes to demon-strate His love to us through other people. This expression refers to a story that is told of a little boy who was afraid of a thunderstorm. When his father comforted him by saying, 'God is with you; you don't have to be afraid,' the little boy responded, 'Yes, I know God loves me, but sometimes it's nice to have people with skin on to give me a hug.'"

Because of the loving responses of all these dear people at a time when I was very vulnerable, I now have a vivid picture in my heart of what love looks like. I have seen God's love at work in a thousand small ways, both in my own heart and through the people around me. As it says in the prayer of Jabez,[16] God has been at work enlarging the territory of my heart, and now I can finally love others.

Sometimes, I still wonder if my contributions to people make any difference at all, but then I remember how good it felt when a friend

---

15   See Ephesians 3:20.
16   1 Chronicles 4:10 (New King James Version): "Oh that you would bless me indeed, and enlarge my territory, that your hand would be with me, and that you would keep me from evil, that I may not cause pain!"

simply looked happy to see me. I know that my ability to love others has its roots in knowing I am loved and also in believing that I am a person of worth who has something good to offer others. I am learning to let my love relationship with God manifest in an outflowing of love to the people around me. And I am learning that it's not necessary to do or say anything—it's enough to just be the person God created and loves.

Being that person is easier said than done. Although He loves me eternally and unconditionally just the way I am, He also sees everything I could be. He points me in new directions and arranges things such that I cannot refuse to go that way if I want to be happy.

Indwelling sin is determined to get me off God's path and onto its own path of destruction by trying to convince me to indulge in my flesh and fears; but God is just as determined to teach me to live life more deeply, genuinely, and fearlessly. Thankfully, God is sovereign and almighty and I know He will win. Philippians 2:6 says, "He who began a good work in you will carry it on to completion."

All my life I had lofty dreams that always came to nothing. As a child, I wanted to play the piano, but I never wanted to practice. I always wanted to learn things, but I never had the self-discipline to study. I always wanted to be loved, but I was never willing to be vulnerable enough to let people into my life. Whenever I did achieve something, I crowed about it to the world and built it up in my mind as a memorial to my greatness. I never knew how to graciously and humbly receive kudos for my good performances. And my successes were few and far between and didn't last very long.

But God had a plan for my life, and He never gave up on me. My cancer journey taught me how to trust that people really do love me and that it really is okay to be me. I just had to surrender to Him. My surrender to His plan for my cancer treatment was a picture of the attitude He wants from me all the time. It was a microcosm of death to my own agenda and living instead to fulfill God's agenda for my life.

The February after my cancer diagnosis, I was introduced to con-templative prayer, sometimes called basking in His presence or silent prayer. (See the bibliography for two excellent books on this subject.) This practice creates in my heart a quiet place where I can always hear His voice, as well as an attitude of surrender. He no longer has to wrestle me to the ground to get me to obey Him. When He speaks, His words instantly become what I want to do.

I still have a long way to go, of course. But an important lesson I have learned is to enjoy the journey rather than waiting to be happy until I reach the destination. The journey is an exciting walk with God through all the paths of life that help me get to know Him better.

I invite you to join me in this journey. Regardless of the circumstances of our lives on this earth, doing things His way guarantees purpose, joy, and overwhelming victory.

Our Deepest Fear
By Marieanne Williamson

Our deepest fear is not that we are inadequate. Our deepest fear is that we are powerful beyond measure. It is our light, not our darkness that most frightens us. We ask ourselves, Who am I to be brilliant, gorgeous, talented, fabulous? Actually, who are you *not* to be? You are a child of God. Your playing small does not serve the world. There is nothing enlightened about shrinking so that other people won't feel insecure around you. We are all meant to shine, as children do. We were born to make manifest the glory of God that is within us. It's not just in some of us; it's in everyone. And as we let our own light shine, we unconsciously give other people permission to do the same. As we are liberated from our own fear, our presence automatically liberates others.[17]

17 Williamson, Marianne. *A Return To Love*. New York, New York: HarperCollins Publishers, Inc., 1992. Used by permission.

Afterword

I am not a qualified medical doctor, and the following is not a prescription for dealing with cancer or any other illness. I thought you might like to know some strategies I use in my efforts to strengthen my immune system and stay healthy. These are not written in stone—I am constantly learning in this area.

★Hydrogen peroxide. After my cancer diagnosis, I consulted a local chiropractor regarding supplements that would strengthen my immune system so it could do its job of killing cancer cells. He suggested adding ten drops of 3 percent hydrogen peroxide to a quarter cup of nonchlorinated water and drinking it twice a day. The idea is that hydrogen peroxide introduces oxygen to the body, and cancer cannot live in a highly oxygenated environment. When I pointed out that the bottle says not to take it internally, he explained that certainly no one should chugalug it, but ten drops twice a day will not hurt anything.

Dr. Higgins[18] said his mother had bladder cancer and her doctor recommended surgery to cut it out. Dr. Higgins had her take the hydrogen peroxide, and three weeks later, they could no longer find any cancer in her.

★Rebounding stimulates circulation and encourages toxin release. See https://www.reboundair.com/33ways.htm for thirty-three ways rebounding is good for the body. I jump on my rebounder five minutes a day and pass the time reviewing Scripture memory work.

★ Get Vitamin D. About twelve minutes of exposure to sunlight each day is optimum. I have heard that much more than that becomes

---

18   Contact information for Dr. Higgins can be found at www.drmarkhiggins.com/.

harmful. I understand that for the body to benefit from sunlight's vitamin D, you should not wash for several hours after exposure to sunlight. When I sit in the sun for this purpose, I do it *after* my morning shower.

★I drink four cups of pure water first thing in the morning, then brush my teeth and wait forty-five minutes before eating or drinking anything else. This is supposed to be very good for the body. Recently, I heard that drinking a cup of hot water with fresh lemon juice first thing in the morning and before bedtime helps the body achieve a proper pH balance, which is extremely important for good health. In the morning, I use part of those four cups of water for my hot lemon water and drink the rest while I wait for the water to heat. I usually use that forty-five minutes for my quiet time with the Lord.

★ Stay positive and live life. Talk over any doubts or negative thoughts with God, give Him those cares, and trust Him completely for the outcome.

★Basking in God's presence. I generally spend twenty minutes a day during my forty-five-minute quiet time being still and silent in God's presence. I have found that this creates a well of quietness within me where I can hear God's voice the rest of the day. It also seems to help me respond to Him more readily. (See bibliography for two excellent books on this topic.)

★Fruit and veggie smoothies. I eat as much of a vegetarian diet as I can manage: minimal meat, lots of fruits and veggies, very little animal fat. For meat, I eat mainly fish or chicken. These smoothies help me get fruit and veggies that I would probably not eat any other way. I started making these smoothies two or three years before my cancer diagnosis.

I make my fruit and veggie smoothies with a Vita Mix[19] blender, a

---

19 See www.vitamix.com/ for information on the Vita Mix. I also recently heard about the Nutribullet that does the same kind of thing. It is much less

powerful appliance that effortlessly purees all parts of the fruit or veggie. This way I get all the nutrients and fiber. I do not know if a regular blender would work as well.

Fruit Smoothie

2 cups strawberries	2 cups grapes
1 can unsweetened pineapple chunks, undrained	1 orange, peeled
1 Granny Smith apple, unpeeled	1 pear, nectarine, or other fruit, pitted, unpeeled

Add all to Vita Mix. Puree thoroughly on high.

Veggie Smoothie

8–9 tomatoes, cored and quartered	4–8 cucumbers, sliced thickly
1 red cabbage, chopped coarsely, cored	1 bunch parsley, chopped in thirds crosswise
1 bunch kale, chopped in thirds crosswise	1 parsnip, cut in 1–2" pieces
6 green, red, and/or yellow peppers, seeded and chopped coarsely	2 heads broccoli with stems, chopped coarsely
1 bunch celery, cut in 1–2" pieces	3–4 beets, scrubbed, chopped coarsely
1 lb. baby carrots	fresh ginger root, washed and cut in 1" pieces

3 lemons, peeled and quartered
3–4 serrano peppers, chopped
brussels sprouts, washed

Add a little of each veggie to the Vita Mix along with one to two cups of water. Puree and pour into a large pitcher. Repeat until all

expensive, but it is also smaller, with only about a two-cup capacity. Check it out at www.nutribullet.com/.

veggies are pureed. If you use the amounts of veggies recommended above, this makes about thirty pounds of veggie smoothie at a cost of about thirty-five dollars. Very cost-effective nutrition! I pour this mixture into sixteen-ounce plastic containers with lids and freeze them. I always have three of these containers defrosting in the refrigerator to mix with a fresh fruit smoothie. This mixture will stay fresh in the refrigerator for several days.

Combine two parts veggie smoothie with one part fruit smoothie.

The fruit smoothie by itself is sweet and tasty. I don't think the veggie smoothie is all that tasty, but it's not bad. Mixing it with the fruit smoothie helps. I drink about sixteen ounces of the fruit and veggie smoothie a day. It is very tasty and filling when mixed with protein powder—I use a chocolate-flavored protein powder from Melaleuca.[20] I would probably never eat things like kale, cabbage, parsley, parsnips, or brussels sprouts if I didn't have them in my smoothies.

My friend, Marguerite, gave me the recipe for this liver cleanse soon after my diagnosis. It is very easy to make.

• •

Fermented Beets for Liver Cleanse

I add a quarter cup of this liquid to my breakfast fruit/veggie/protein powder smoothie, along with a quarter cup of Kefir and one tablespoon of raw, organic, unfiltered, apple cider vinegar.

1 qt. yogurt, unsweetened, full fat, plain
2 fresh beets, unpeeled, scrubbed, cut into ¼" slices
1 tablespoon sea salt dissolved in water

Drain yogurt overnight in a wire sieve in refrigerator. The drained part is whey—you can store it in a glass jar in the refrigerator for six months. Put a quarter cup of whey and the beets in a two-quart jar, add

---

20   See www.melaleuca.com/ or e-mail me at grangle@q.com for more information about this excellent company.

salt dissolved in water, and add water to fill jar. Cover jar and keep on kitchen counter for two days to ferment. Then strain off the liquid and drink a quarter cup morning and night to gently cleanse the liver.

After the two days of fermenting at room temperature, store in refrigerator.

For second batch from the same whey: When the liquid is almost gone, leave a half cup of liquid in the jar and remove beets. You can eat the beets at this point—they are *very* good for you in this form. I puree them and add them to my veggie smoothies. Add one tablespoon of sea salt dissolved in water and two fresh beets (prepared as above) to the jar. Fill the jar and ferment for two more days.

Resources

www.drmarkhiggins.com/ for contact information about Dr. Higgins, who suggested the hydrogen peroxide protocol.

http://jonathantreasure.com/ for the herbalist with whom I consulted.

http://www.mederifoundation.org/ for the clinic in Oregon from which I ordered my supplements.

See http://www.melaleuca.com/ or e-mail me at grangle@q.com for more information about this excellent company that offers safe and effective supplements, shakes, cleaning supplies, and beauty products for reasonable prices.

http://www.mylifeline.org/ and http://www.caringbridge.org/ are websites specifically for sharing one's cancer journey with friends and family.

http://www.nutribullet.com/ for information on the Nutribullet.

www.vitamix.com/ for information on the Vita Mix.

References

Scripture

1 Chronicles 4:10 (New King James Version) – Prayer of Jabez.

Daniel 3:13–27 – the story of Shadrach, Meshach, and Abednego in the fiery furnace.

Romans 2:1 – In whatever you judge another you condemn yourself.

Romans 6:11 – Die to sin and live only to God.

Romans 7:17 – On indwelling sin.

Romans 8:28 – All things work together for the good of those who love Him.

2 Corinthians 10:3–6 and Ephesians 6:10–18 – On spiritual warfare.

Ephesians 3:20 – We can't even imagine everything God has in store for us.

Ephesians 5:20 – Being thankful for all things.

Revelation 12:10 – Satan is the accuser of the brethren.

Books and Web Pages

Arnold, Veronica, August 2, 2011, blog entry, http://www.mylife-line.org/.

Harris, Jan. *Quiet in His Presence: Experiencing God's Love through Silent Prayer.* Grand Rapids, Michigan: Baker Books, 2003.

Oldielyrics. Lyrics to "Then You Can Tell Me Goodbye" by John D. Loudermill, accessed August 2, 2012, http://www.oldielyrics.com/lyrics/the_casinos/then_you_can_tell_me_goodbye.html.

Pierce, Tanya Harter. *Outsmart Your Cancer: Alternative Non-Toxic*

Treatments That Work. Stateline, Nevada: Thoughtworks Publishing 2004.

Quinn, Hollie and Patrick. *You Did What? Saying "No" to Conventional Cancer Treatment.* Cobblestone Publishing, LLC, 2010.

Volkman, Bill. *Basking in His Presence: A Call to the Prayer of Silence.* Glen Ellyn, Illinois: Union Life Ministries, 1996.

Williamson, Marianne. *A Return To Love.* New York, New York: HarperCollins Publishers, Inc., 1992. Used by permission.

About the Author

Veronica Arnold lives in Fort Collins, Colorado, with her husband. Their two adult children live nearby with their families and assorted pets. Veronica worked as a rural-route mail carrier for the US Postal Service for thirty years. Presently she works at home as a biblical counselor/lay minister. After completing a two-year course in preparation for that work, she began working toward a degree in counseling, taking classes at Front Range Community College in Fort Collins. She is director of the Mercy Ministry at her church, Iasis Christ Fellowship, in Fort Collins.